Man Ma

Challenges & Choices

Contents

Challenges & Choices 3
Booze 4
Food 8
Exercise 13
Sexually-transmitted infections 15
Local health services 17
Blood pressure 18
Stress 21
Tobacco 24
Skin 27
Back 29

© Ian Banks 2009

(019-12409)

ISBN: 978 1 906121 80 8

All rights reserved. No part of this booklet may be reproduced or transmitted in any form or by any means, electronic or mechanical, including photocopying, recording or by any information storage or retrieval system, without permission in writing from the copyright holder.

Printed in the UK.

Haynes Publishing, Sparkford, Yeovil, Somerset BA22 7JJ, England

Haynes North America, Inc, 861 Lawrence Drive, Newbury Park, California 91320, USA

Haynes Publishing Nordiska AB, Box 1504, 751 45 Uppsala, Sweden

The Author and the Publisher have taken care to ensure that the advice given in this edition is current at the time of publication. The Reader is advised to read and understand the instructions and information material included with all medicines recommended, and to consider carefully the appropriateness of any treatments. The Author and the Publisher will have no liability for adverse results, inappropriate or excessive use of the remedies offered in this book or their level of effectiveness in individual cases. The Author and the Publisher do not intend that this book be used as a substitute for medical advice. Advice from a medical practitioner should always be sought for any symptom or illness.

2 MAN MANUAL – CHALLENGES & CHOICES

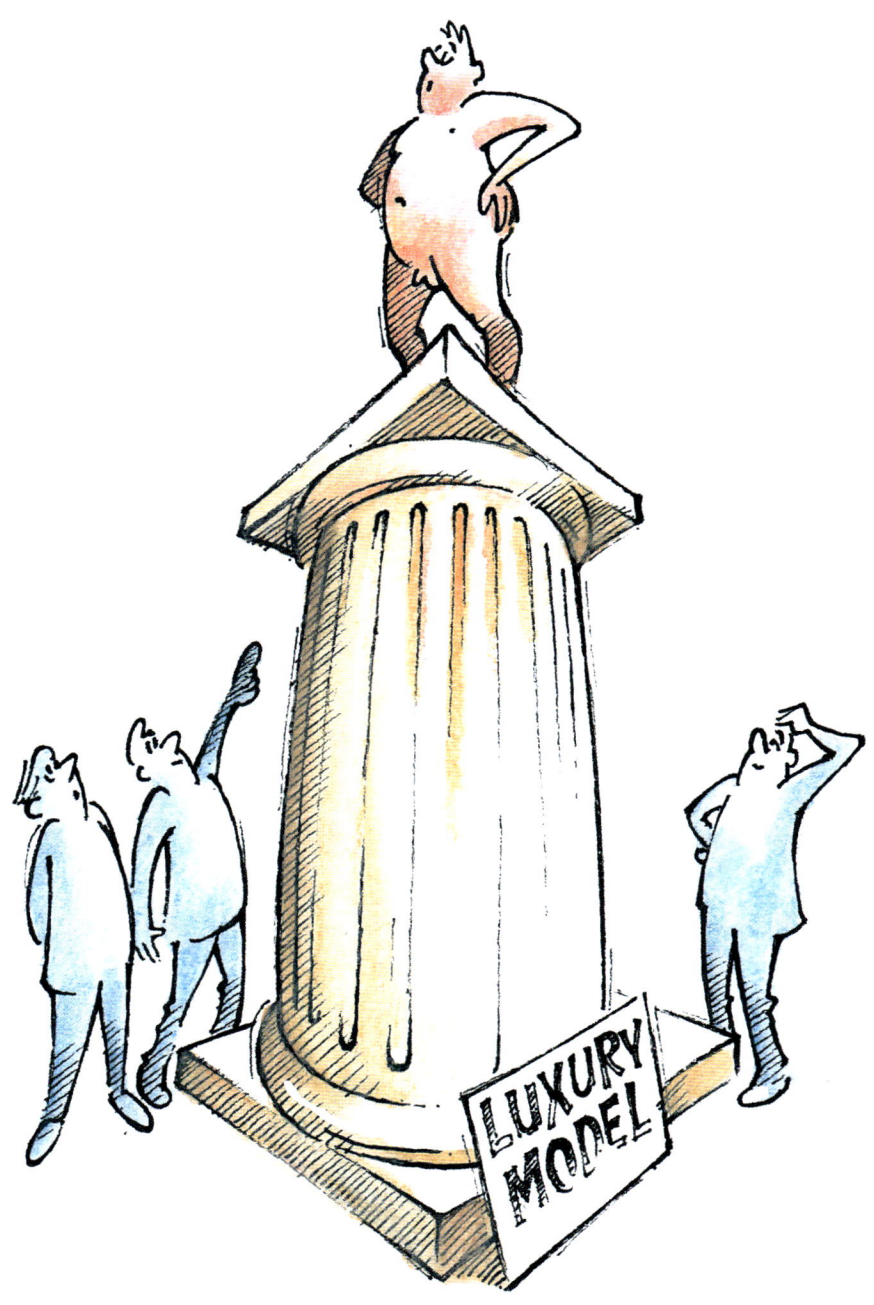

Challenges & Choices

Here is your first challenge: Read this manual

Don't worry, it won't ask you to do the impossible. There is no shortage of people queuing up to tell you just exactly what you must do to improve your health. Unfortunately most don't ask what you *want to do*.

So, just for a change, to meet every challenge we give you three choices. The first choice is to do nothing, just like when the warning light on the dashboard comes on and you choose to keep driving until you need a new engine. The second choice is DIY (so when the warning light comes on, you stop and check the oil level). The third choice is to find an expert.

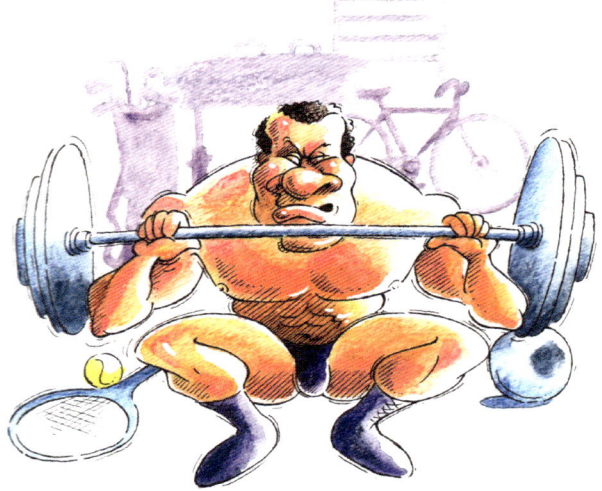

Check out

www.malehealth.co.uk

Fast, free independent health info for men. News, features, an online gym and your fitness questions answered.

It's up to you, but are you up for it?

4 MAN MANUAL – CHALLENGES & CHOICES

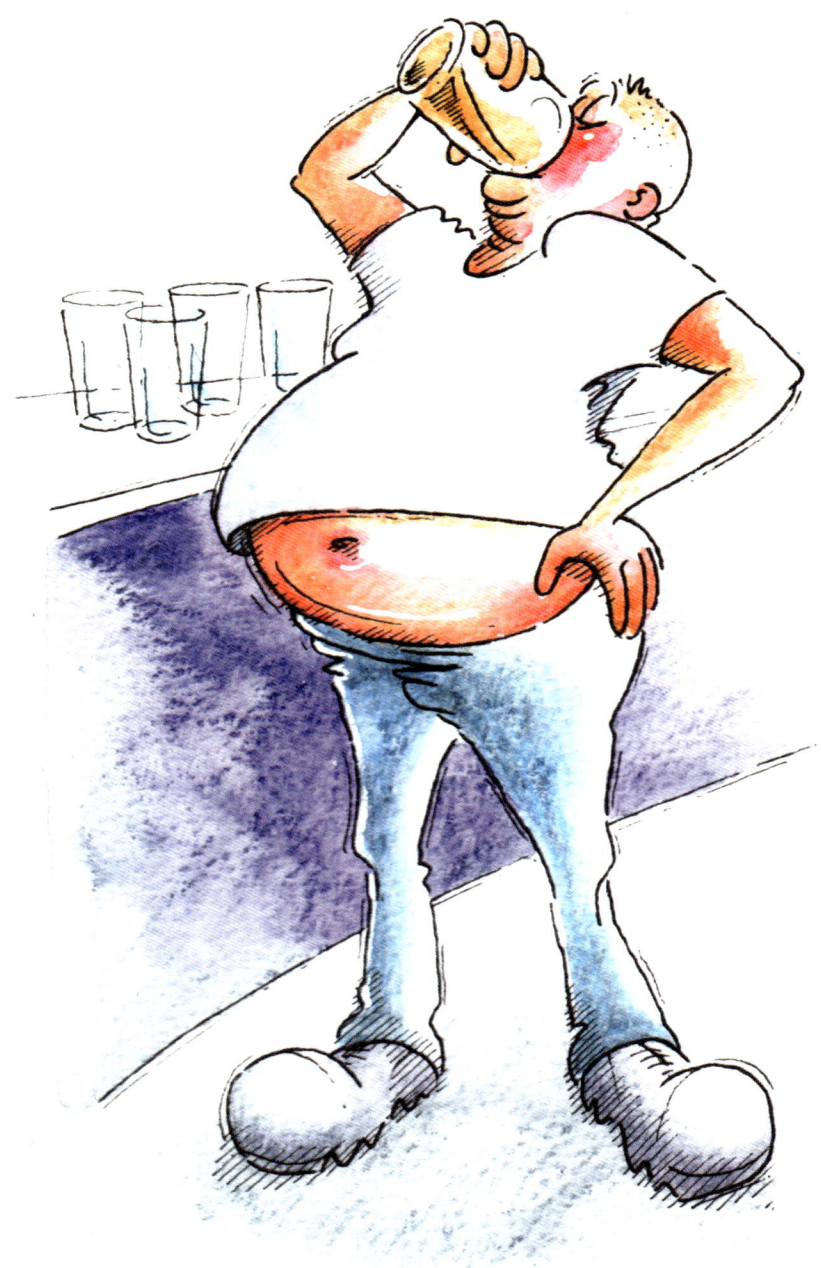

Booze

The Challenge

Order a soft drink next time you're in the pub.

The Reason

A round or two (or three or four if it's Friday) with your workmates may seem a good way of rounding off the working day. Wine with a meal also probably improves digestion, not to mention conversation!

The problems start if you drink too much and too often. Three in ten men are drinking in ways that could damage their health in the future. If you regularly drink more than 3 to 4 units of alcohol a day (4 units are two pints of normal lager, one and a half of strong lager, or half a bottle of wine) you are risking your health.

Since the 1970s there has been an eight-fold increase in deaths from chronic liver disease amongst men aged 35 to 44. One in six people attending Accident and Emergency has alcohol-related injuries or problems – and this rises to eight in ten at peak times. Around 20% of psychiatric hospital admissions are alcohol-related.

At work, accidents (sometimes fatal) are more common in the afternoon after lunchtime drinks. More than half of all fatal car accidents, falls and drownings are alcohol-related.

The Choices

Do nothing
OK, but around 16 men die of alcohol problems every day in the UK. It might be your round next.

DIY
Some simple steps you can take to continue enjoying your evenings at the pub whilst avoiding the harmful effects.
- Walk to the pub and burn off some of the extra calories on the way.
- Drink plenty of water before, during and after the pub. If you're thirsty, you'll tend to drink more alcohol.
- Drink after a meal rather than before; you won't feel so hungry and so won't feel like drinking so much.
- Cut down the strength of your drinks. If you normally drink strong lager (5% ABV), try switching to a normal lager (3.5% ABV).
- Try to have one alcohol-free day each week – and if you can manage that, then go for two or three.

Avoid mixing alcohol and work. As already pointed out, not only does the lunchtime pint impair work performance and increase your chances of an accident in the afternoon, it also uses up some of your precious 'maximum units'.

UNITS

The currently accepted recommended maximum weekly intake for men is 21 units (and 14 units for women). Major problems become much more likely with a weekly intake of over 35 units for men (and over 21 units for women).

The number of units of alcohol in a drink depends on the amount (volume) and strength (ABV).

- Small glass of wine (125ml) at 12% ABV = 1½ units.
- Large glass of wine (175ml) at 15% ABV = 3 units.
- Bottle of wine (750ml) at 12% ABV = 9 units.
- Bottle of wine (750ml) at 15% ABV = 12 units.
- Pint of beer at 3.5% ABV = 2 units.
- Pint of beer at 5% ABV = 3 units.
- Single measure of spirits (25ml) at 40% ABV = 1 unit.

AT HOME

If you do most of your drinking at home rather than at the pub, the same general advice applies, but there are some particular points to think about:
- If you drink spirits, watch your measures. Pouring freehand generally results in a larger measure than you get in the pub.
- When buying beer or wine to take home, choose those with the lower alcohol content. A bottle of wine between two with a meal may not seem like much, but if it's 15% ABV that's 6 units each.

Find an expert

If you are worried about your drinking, sources of further help and advice include:
- Your GP, who will be able to advise you further, check out your physical health, and can put you in touch with local sources of help.
- Give NHS Direct a ring or go online.

NHS Direct
Tel: 0845 4647 (24 hour service)
www.nhsdirect.nhs.uk

Alcohol Concern
Has a useful website, with a services directory for information on how to access local alcohol services across the UK.
www.alcoholconcern.org.uk

Alcoholics Anonymous
Tel: 0845 769 7555 (local rate calls)

Drinkaware
Tel: 0207 307 7450
www.drinkaware.co.uk

Drinkline
Offers information and self-help materials, help to callers worried about their own drinking, support to the family and friends of people who are drinking, and advice to callers on where to go for help.
Tel: 0800 917 8282 (freephone)

www.malehealth.co.uk/drinking

Food

The Challenge

Try some fruit or veg you've never tasted before or think you don't like.

The Reason

A well-balanced diet not only improves your general health and well-being and helps maintain a healthy weight, but can also lower your blood cholesterol, keep your blood pressure down, and reduce your risk of developing heart disease, diabetes and some cancers.

The Choices

Do nothing

Around 9 out of 10 blokes don't eat enough fruit and veg. Much the pity. Heart disease is the single biggest man killer and over 16,000 people in the UK will die from bowel cancer each year. Both can be prevented.

DIY

First of all, do actually have breakfast. You wouldn't expect your car to work without fuel, and your body is no different. Equally, you wouldn't put

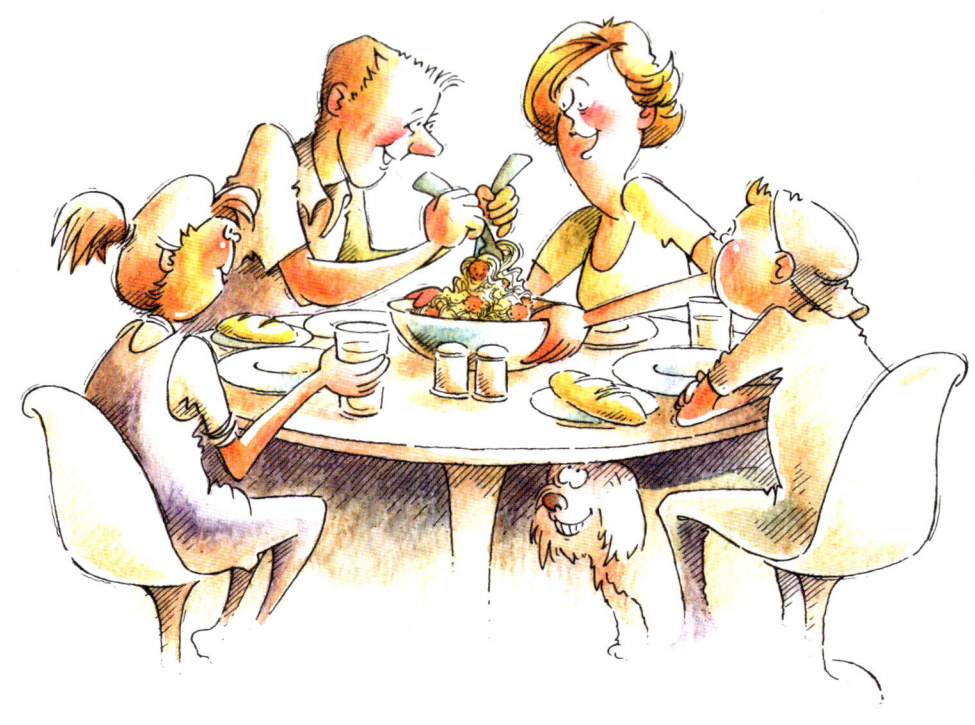

MAN MANUAL – CHALLENGES & CHOICES

crude oil in your car, so take care over what you eat. That traditional fried breakfast may be tempting – and once in a while won't harm you – but did you know that a typical fry-up with bacon, sausages, fried egg, toast and a dollop of sauce is going to take up half your recommended daily intake of calories, almost all your total and saturated fat allowance, just about your entire salt intake and most of your daily protein as well?

If you like a cooked breakfast, why not try beans on toast, or scrambled eggs and mushrooms on toast – but make the toast wholemeal and grill rather than fry those mushrooms!

Or maybe try some of the following instead:

- A cereal with no added sugar, preferably wholegrain and low in salt. Perhaps try with skimmed or semi-skimmed milk.
- Some fruit.
- A couple of slices of wholemeal toast with margarine (or at least low-salt butter).
- A medium-sized glass of fruit drink – either fruit juice (not squash – which doesn't count towards the 5-a-day quota) or a fruit smoothie.

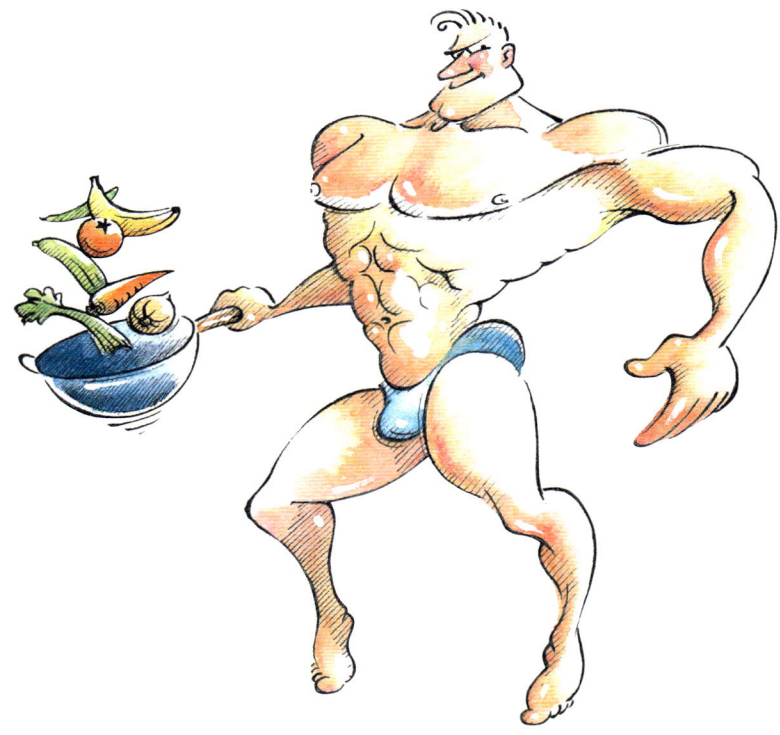

It's easy to build at least

5

different fruit and veg into your day.

One portion is:

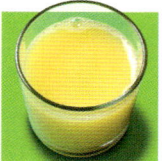
1 medium glass of orange juice

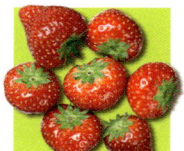
7 strawberries

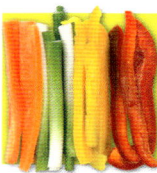
A handful of sliced peppers, onions and carrots

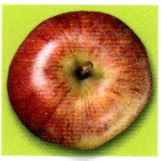
1 medium apple

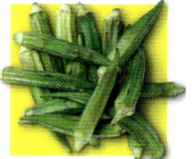
16 okra

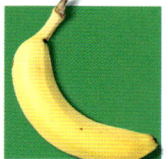
1 medium banana

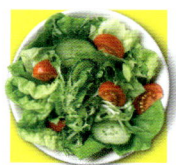
1 small mixed salad

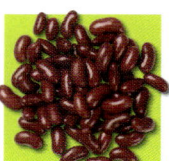
3 heaped tablespoons of cooked kidney beans

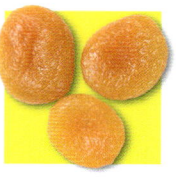
3 whole dried apricots

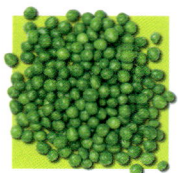
3 heaped tablespoons of peas

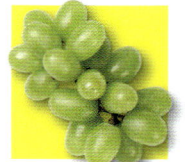
1 handful of grapes

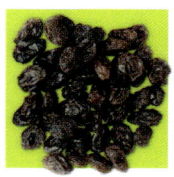
1 tablespoon raisins

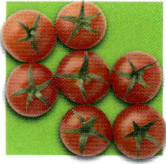
7 cherry tomatoes

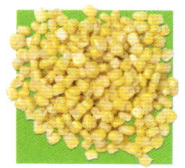
3 heaped tablespoons of corn

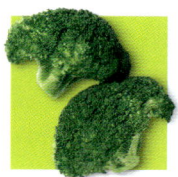
2 spears of broccoli

Fruit and vegetables

Unless you have been hiding under a rock for the past few years, you will know that eating plenty of fruit and vegetables every day is vital for great health. The average guide is to eat at least five servings each day (equivalent to 400 g). Almost all fruit and vegetables count towards your five servings a day. What's more there's no limit to how much you can consume – so the more you eat, the better. It's also good to know that you should eat a variety of fruit and vegetables to get the maximum nutritional benefits. This is because they each contain different combinations of fibre, vitamins, minerals and other nutrients. Besides, eating the same ones every day would be boring.

Reaching 5-a-day doesn't have to be difficult or unpleasant. Consider the following:
- A handful of raisins on your cereal in the morning is not only tasty – but counts as one.
- A glass of OJ and you're at two already.
- An apple will give you more long-term energy than a cup of coffee.
- Copy your favourite tennis player and grab a banana for extra energy.
- Chop up lots of vegetables and use them in a stir-fry. Quick, easy and super healthy.
- Add some mushrooms or peas in your curry – and you've hit 6-a-day. Easy Peasy!

Starchy foods

You also need to make sure you have enough starchy foods in your diet. Most men should be eating:
- More bread, especially wholemeal or granary breads, but also seedy bread, chapattis, pitta bread, bagels and tortillas.
- More foods such as rice, pasta (wholegrain varieties where possible) and potatoes (but not chips).
- More beans, lentils or peas.

Fat in your diet

Watch the fat in your diet. You should be cutting down on food that is high in saturated fat or trans fats which can increase the amount of cholesterol in the blood and increase the risk of developing heart disease.

Foods to avoid include:
- Meat products, such as meat pies and sausages.
- Fast food.
- Hard cheese, butter and lard.
- Some margarines.
- Pastry, cakes and biscuits.
- Cream, coconut oil and palm oil.

Consider replacing these with foods high in unsaturated fat which actually reduce cholesterol levels, as well as providing essential fatty acids. Foods high in unsaturated fats are:
- Oily fish (such as sardines or mackerel).
- Avocados.
- Nuts and seeds.
- Sunflower, rapeseed, olive and vegetable oils (and spreads).

Salt in your diet

It's also important to cut down the amount of salt in your diet. Although salt is vital for life, too much is harmful as it can raise your blood pressure. People with high blood pressure are three times more likely to develop heart disease or have a stroke than those with normal blood pressure.

Ways to reduce salt include:
- Eating home-cooked meals wherever possible.
- Using fresh or frozen vegetables rather than canned ones.
- Eating fresh poultry, fish or lean meat, rather than smoked or processed types.
- Cooking rice, pasta and vegetables without salt.
- Cutting back on frozen dinners, pizza, instant rice and pasta, canned soups and salad dressings.
- Avoiding foods preserved in brine (such as pickled vegetables) and condiments (such as mustard and ketchup, and barbecue sauce).

Find an expert

Good advice and support from:

5-A-DAY
Tel: 0207 210 4850
www.5aday.nhs.uk

British Heart Foundation
14 Fitzhardinge Street
London
W1H 6DH
Tel: 020 7935 0185
www.bhf.org.uk

Cholesterol UK
35 Bedford Row
London
WC1R 4JH
Tel: 0207 400 4480
www.cholesteroluk.org.uk

Diabetes UK
Tel: 0845 120 2960
www.diabetes.org.uk

Food Standards Agency
Tel: 0207 276 8000
www.eatwell.gov.uk

H•E•A•R•T UK
Tel: 0845 450 5988
www.heartuk.org.uk

National Heart Forum
Tavistock House South
Tavistock Square
London
WC1H 9LG
Tel: 020 7383 7638
www.heartforum.org.uk

www.malehealth.co.uk/diet

Exercise

The Challenge

Make at least one journey by foot or bicycle instead of going by car.

The Reason

Around 100,000 men die early each and every year in the UK. That's one man every four and a half minutes. Some men can run a mile in under that time.

The Choices

Do nothing

Lack of physical activity together with poor diet has led to more than 1 in 5 men in England now being obese. A further 40% are overweight. Diabetes caused by obesity is increasing fast. Diabetes is one of the single most common causes of erectile dysfunction (ED or impotence). Being up for it may be a bigger problem than you think.

DIY

Men who increase their activity level over a five year period cut their chances of dying early by almost half. Walking instead of using the car helps your health, your bank balance and the environment.

Exercise will make you feel better, make you look better and who knows… maybe even make you more

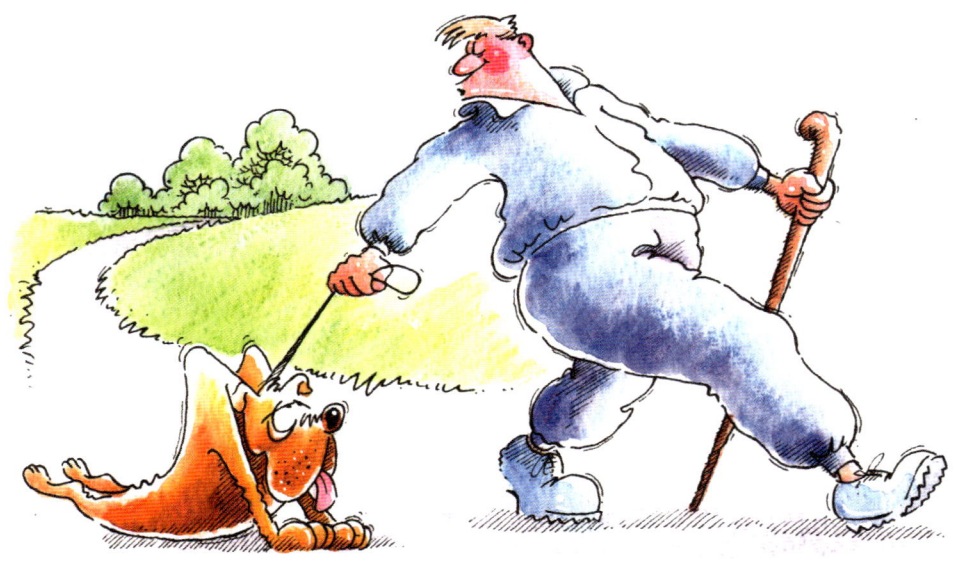

attractive (showers permitting of course!).

Of course many jobs require a significant amount of exercise. But if your job doesn't, there are simple things you can consider doing to make exercise part of your normal working day. And what better way to start than with the journey to work in the morning.

Travelling to and from work
The journey to work is an ideal chance to help build up the 30 minutes a day of regular physical activity you need. It also has added benefits, as you could save on petrol, fares and commuter stress.

Walking or cycling to work (or to the train station if you have a longer journey), instead of driving or using public transport, could make a huge difference. If it takes you 15 minutes each way, you would immediately achieve your recommended daily amount of exercise – and it may even take less time than battling through the traffic.

If your employer doesn't already have schemes in place ask them if they can help encourage walking and cycling to work.

At work
There are a number of simple things you can do during the work day to stay active – and remember the little things add up!

- Take the stairs instead of the lift; if you work on the top floor get off a few floors early.
- Take opportunities to walk around the office: deliver documents or messages to co-workers in person rather than by email
- Go for a walk at lunch time and during breaks.
- Maybe join a sports team for lunch-time or after work.

Find an expert

National Obesity Forum
Tel: 0115 846 2329
www.nationalobesityforum.org.uk

Sport England
Tel: 0207 273 1551
www.sportengland.org

Sport Scotland
Tel: 0131 317 7200
www.sportscotland.org.uk

Sports Council Wales
Tel: 0845 045 0904
www.sports-council-wales.org.uk

Sustrans
Tel: 0845 113 0065
www.sustrans.org.uk

Weight Concern
Tel: 0207 679 6639
www.weightconcern.org.uk

www.malehealth.co.uk/exercise

Sexually-transmitted infections

The Challenge

If you're under 25 and sexually active, get yourself checked for chlamydia, the most common sexually-transmitted infection.

The Reason

Chlamydia isn't a Greek island or an edible shell fish – it's actually the UK's most common sexually-transmitted infection and getting worse. There are often no symptoms so you won't know you've got it (until you want to have a kid and you or your partner aren't able to).

The Choices

Do nothing

You might never know if you are infected but your female partners will soon find out when they suffer from the commonest cause of infertility and are unable to have children or suffer a baby developing in the wrong part of their body (ectopic pregnancy). But then, hey, that's their problem, so that's OK (isn't it?).

DIY

Just one tip for preventing sexually-transmitted infections: always practise safer sex. No ifs or buts. Use a condom whenever you have sex, because to be honest sexually-transmitted infections are a great leveller. They can affect you at any age, whether you're straight or gay, in a long-term relationship or with a casual partner. Symptoms don't always show up immediately, so you could have been infected recently or a long time ago.

Although extra lubrication is sometimes required, do not use oil-based lubricants such as petroleum jelly or baby oil. They will damage most types of condom. There are water-based lubricants available. If you are not sure, ask the chemist; they will not be embarrassed to give advice.

DOES TAKING THE PILL PROTECT YOU FROM STIs?

STI stands for Sexually Transmitted Infection. The Pill most definitely does not stop women picking up fellow travellers. Condoms on the other hand will protect you and your partner from almost all nether region nasties and prevent unwanted pregnancies. Unfortunately, men will often leave contraception all up to the woman. Vaginal condoms are now available which really do protect a woman from a fate worse than death, in fact just death.

Find an expert

All well and good to say use a condom but mistakes do happen especially when the spirit is 40% and the flesh is willing. You might not always know you have an infection but a simple test will. Even so watch out for any discharge from the penis. A one-off dose of antibiotic does the trick for chlamydia.

If you haven't practised safe sex or are at all worried, you can have a confidential check-up, and treatment if needed, at a genitourinary medicine (GUM) or STI clinic. Call NHS Direct for details of your nearest clinic.

NHS Direct
Tel: 0845 4647 (24 hour service)
www.nhsdirect.nhs.uk

Brook
Tel: 08000 185 023
www.brook.org.uk

National Chlamydia Screening Programme
Tel: 0800 567 123
www.chlamydiascreening.nhs.uk

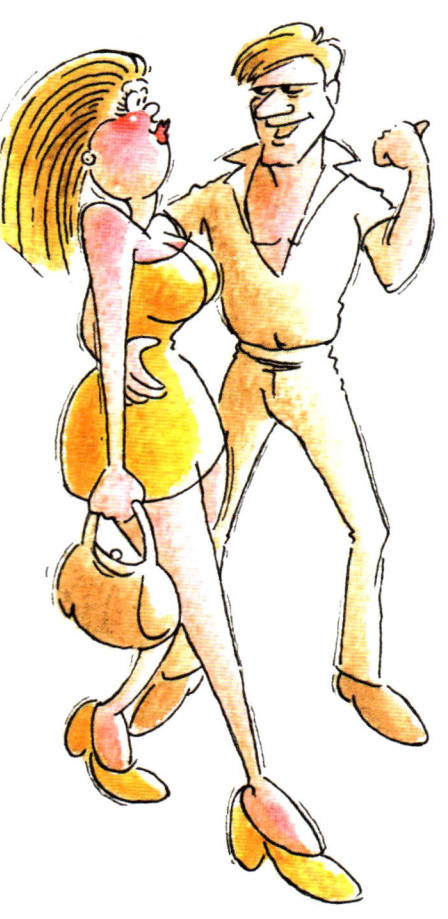

www.malehealth.co.uk/sexualhealth

MAN MANUAL – CHALLENGES & CHOICES **17**

Local health services

The Challenge

Find out the opening hours at your local GP's surgery (and register as a patient if you haven't already).

The Reason

Men use primary care much less than women and tend to wait until things have got really bad before finally turning up. No wonder then that for every cancer both men and women suffer, men come off worse. Remember, primary care includes the local pharmacy and walk-in centres.

While you are there, get your blood pressure checked. It might help you avoid a heart attack or stroke.

The Choices

Do nothing

Sounds reasonable, but sticking your head in the sand isn't going to make any problems go away.

DIY

If you have a well-stocked, locked medicines box at home, you may be able to deal with the problem yourself. Useful medicines include paracetamol and ibuprofen 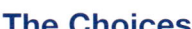 for pain, fever and headaches, antihistamines for allergies and hay fever, and indigestion remedy for heartburn and trapped wind. Ask your pharmacist about which medicines to keep at home.

Remember – if you are unsure you can call NHS Direct.

Find an expert

NHS Direct
Tel: 0845 4647 (24 hour service)
www.nhsdirect.nhs.uk

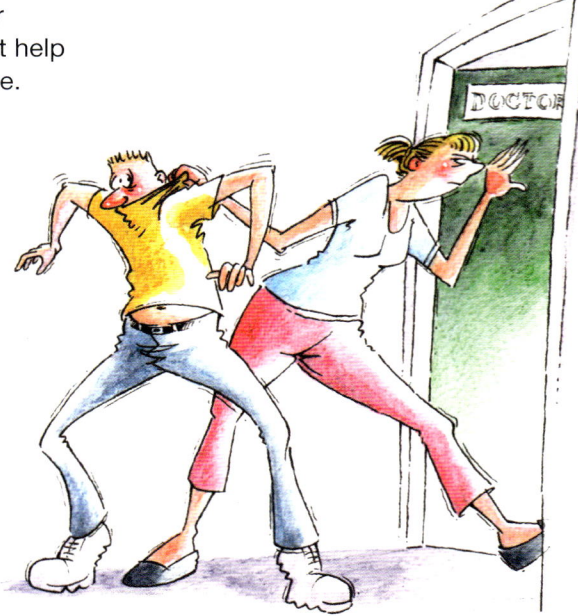

www.malehealth.co.uk/nhs

Blood pressure

The Challenge

Get your blood pressure checked within the next two weeks.

The Reason

High blood pressure (hypertension) is rightly called the 'Silent Killer' because there are very few signs that things are going horribly wrong. Only by measuring your blood pressure will you know if you are in danger. A car tyre can look perfectly fine yet may be at a dangerous pressure.

Blood pressure varies throughout the day. This is normal, and occurs in everyone, whether they have high blood pressure or not. Blood pressure responds to activity or rest. As you get older blood pressure tends to rise. High blood pressure is also more common among people of African-Caribbean descent. Diabetes and other illnesses are also associated with raised blood pressure.

When your blood pressure is measured, it is done when the heart beats (systolic pressure) and when the heart relaxes between beats (diastolic pressure). Both pressures are measured in millimetres of mercury, written as 'mmHg', and when blood pressure is measured and recorded, the systolic reading is always written before the diastolic figure. High blood pressure is defined as a consistent blood pressure over 140/90 mm but there are doctors who feel even this is too high.

Why is high blood pressure dangerous?

High blood pressure puts a strain on blood vessels all over the body, including vital arteries to the brain. The excess pressure can damage the lining of an artery, allowing blood clots to form and cause blockages. The extra strain may also cause blood vessels to burst, so that blood spills into surrounding tissues. This is what causes a stroke.

Choices

Do nothing

This is without doubt the easiest option and is very popular with men. Which may explain why stroke is so much higher than in women.

DIY

After seeing your pharmacist or practice nurse, buy a simple blood pressure monitor. They can be bought for as little as £10 and are very good but you should be checked by an expert every six months or so if you have high blood pressure. Check out the stuff on salt in your diet on page 12 as it is one of the major causes of high blood pressure and easy to cut down on. Stop shaking the shaker.

MAN MANUAL – CHALLENGES & CHOICES **19**

Find an expert

There are professionals out there just waiting to wrap a cuff round your arm.

Pharmacists: More than just blue bottles

Pharmacists are highly qualified professionals providing advice on the use and selection of prescription and over-the-counter (OTC) medicines. They are experts at managing minor ailments and common conditions. This includes lifestyle advice not least for nutrition, physical activity and stopping smoking but they will also signpost you to other health and social care services.

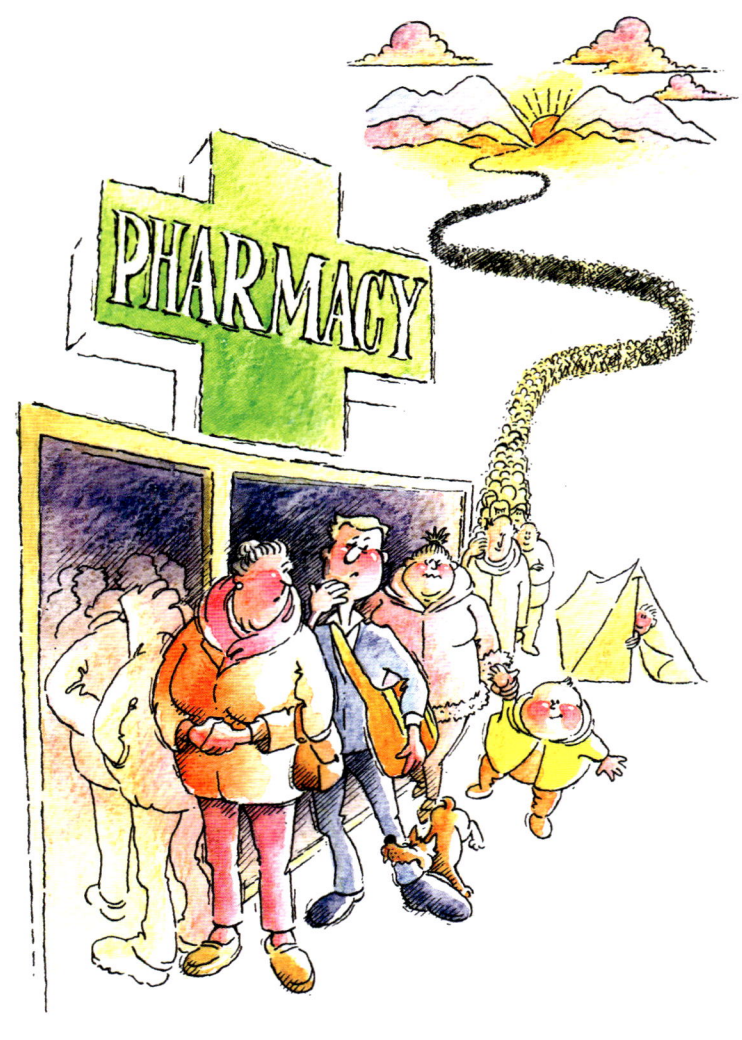

NHS Walk-in Centres: A step in the right direction

Convenient, appointment free and in places where you are. Highly qualified NHS nurses offer a range of services: good advice, care of minor ailments and injuries, prescriptions and even emergency contraception. Look out for the centres in railway stations, shopping malls or on the high street. They generally open from 7 am until 10 pm Monday to Friday, 9 am to 10 pm Saturday and Sunday.

NHS Direct: Direct and to the point

NHS Direct provides 24 hour confidential health advice and information. Call 0845 4647 or visit NHS Direct Online at www.nhsdirect.nhs.uk. And why not try NHS Direct Interactive on digital satellite TV?

GPs: Family medicine

General practitioners are available from around 8.30 am to 6 pm or later. Calling at other times will put you in touch with an out of hours system run by qualified GPs and nurses. It's always best to see your own doctor if possible so unless your need is urgent and cannot wait make an appointment to be seen by your practice GP. Practices now often offer a huge range of services such as minor surgery, skin care, antenatal care and even diabetic clinics (once only provided by hospital out patient departments).

NHS Direct

Tel: 0845 4647 (24 hour service)
www.nhsdirect.nhs.uk

Blood Pressure Association

60 Cranmer Terrace
London
SW17 0QS
Tel: 020 8772 4994
www.bpassoc.org.uk

Salt Campaign – The Food Standards Agency

www.salt.gov.uk

The Stroke Association

240 City Road
London
EC1V 2PR
Helpline: 0845 30 33 100
www.stroke.org.uk

www.malehealth.co.uk/bp

Stress

The Challenge

Stressed out? Walk out before you blow up. Removing yourself from the situation gives you the space to work out the best thing to do.

The Reason

Let's be honest, life without stress is impossible. It can even help you perform better and give you a buzz. But a build-up of pressure without the chance to recover can lead to dangerous stress. Far from being helpful, now it can actually harm your health and even those around you.

Few of us are unfamiliar with feelings of stress such as being worried, tense or feeling unable to cope. But hang on in there, the good news is that there are things you can do to deal with, and manage, stress at home and at work especially with support from family and friends.

Stress signals

Although we all have to deal with stress of some sort ether at work or home, people vary in how much stress they can take before it has an effect on their life.

Watch out for the common stress signals including:
- Eating more or less than normal.
- Mood swings.
- Poor concentration.
- Feeling tense.
- Feeling useless.
- Anxiety.
- Not sleeping properly, especially waking early and not getting back off to sleep.
- Tiredness.
- Poor memory/forgetfulness.

Part of the problem is not recognising our own stress signals and expecting too much of ourselves.

Why bother?

Being stressed can trigger more than common mental health problems like anxiety and depression such as:
- Back pain.
- Indigestion.
- Irritable bowel syndrome.
- Psoriasis.

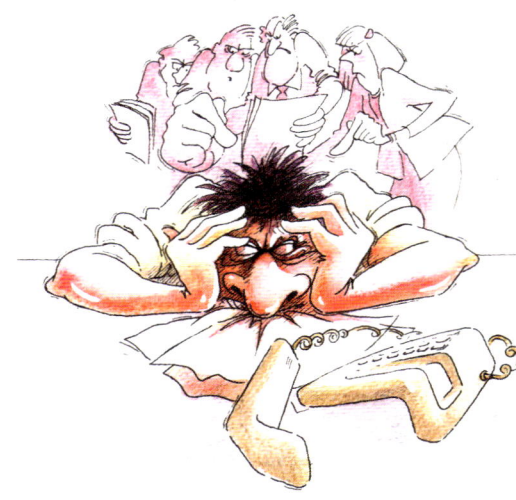

- Migraine.
- Tension headaches.

Thankfully there are several things that you can do to help yourself deal with and prevent stress and to improve how you feel both physically and mentally in the long run.

The Choices

Do nothing
'You Cannot Be Serious'.

DIY

1. Time out
It can be hard to be rational when you are feeling very stressed, which is why it's important to take some time out.
Quick fix
Getting yourself out of a stressful situation, even for a few moments, can give you the space you need to feel more able to tackle the problem. Easy to say but often hard to manage.
Long term
Taking time out from your everyday routine may help you deal with, and avoid, stress. If you have young children it is important to get a break. Try organising a babysitter for an evening, or take it in turns with your partner to have time to yourselves. If you work, try to avoid doing long hours, take proper holidays and take breaks away from your work area each day.

2. Work out
Exercise really helps blow off steam and prevents stress-linked illness.

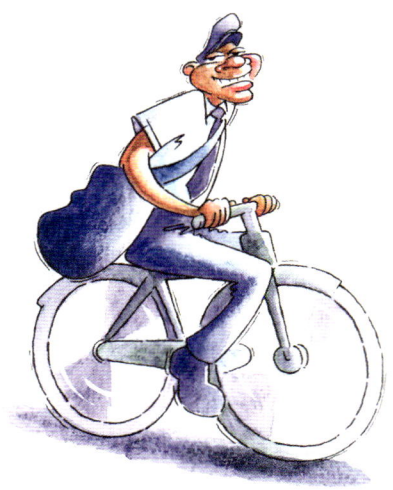

Quick fix
Go for a quick walk round the block – this can help clear your head so you can tackle problems better.
Long term
Go for at least 30 minutes of activity a day. This doesn't have to be done all at once and can be done in bouts of 10 minutes. Try building activity into your daily routine like cycling or walking to the shops, taking stairs instead of lifts, going for a walk and playing games with the children.

3. Chill out
Getting enough sleep as well as relaxing your mind will all help you cope with stress. Avoid sleeping tablets as they can be addictive and make things even worse.
Quick fix
Simple relaxation techniques such as deep breathing can be an effective way of helping you deal with stress.

Long term
Plan time to relax, even if it's just having a long bath or listening to music. Try to have a good night's sleep. Relaxation techniques can be useful for many people in helping them to feel more able to cope. There are many types of relaxation classes available such as meditation, yoga and Pilates.

4. Leave it out
Avoid taking refuge in smoking, junk food or alcohol! This won't help your stress levels. Avoid too many caffeinated and sugary drinks: caffeine may make you feel more anxious and bursts of sugar can cause mood swings.
Quick fix
Drink plenty of water. This will help you concentrate better and may stop you getting stress headaches.
Long term
Improving your diet and drinking plenty of water will increase your body's resistance to stress. It's important to make time for proper meals to help you stay energised. Talk over meals. This is a time to unwind, eat rather than just stuff the neck.

5. Talk it out
Just talking about things that are causing you stress may help you see things in a different light. It can help you find a way forward in tackling practical problems that may be causing you stress.

Talk with friends or family
Going it alone is never a good idea. Even one other person to talk to can help you deal with stress. Talk with family or friends about how you are feeling – they may be able to offer their support.
Talk with colleagues
Hard to believe but work is generally good for our well-being but, at times, it can be stressful. Us men tend not to want to talk about work problems but it might just save your brain power by chatting with your mates.

Most employers these days want to hear of problems before they lose a valuable employee. Trade unions also have people specially trained to deal with workplace stress. If your company has a counselling or occupational health service then use it. They are there to help you and the service is confidential. Research shows that people who experience work-based stress benefit from these services.

Find an expert

Talk with a health professional
You can speak to a GP or practice nurse for advice and support, or contact NHS Direct. You can also ask your pharmacist for advice.

NHS Direct
Tel: 0845 4647 (24 hour service)
www.nhsdirect.nhs.uk

www.malehealth.co.uk/stress

Tobacco

The Challenge

Get a mate to give up smoking with you (if you've already given up, the challenge is to try to stop looking so smug about it).

The Reason

Okay, so you've heard it all before. But don't turn the page yet. This advice could add years to your life, never mind helping to improve the way you look, feel and smell.

Smoking is the single greatest cause of death. Full stop. It has killed more people than both world wars put together. It can also affect your children and those around you. Smoking causes lung cancer – even the tobacco companies now accept this simple fact. It can also lead to all sorts of serious health problems, including heart disease, stroke, various other cancers (such as bladder, mouth and throat cancers), in addition to bronchitis and emphysema.

But OK enough of the bad news, check this out: what you may not know is that the very moment you stop smoking your health will start to improve.

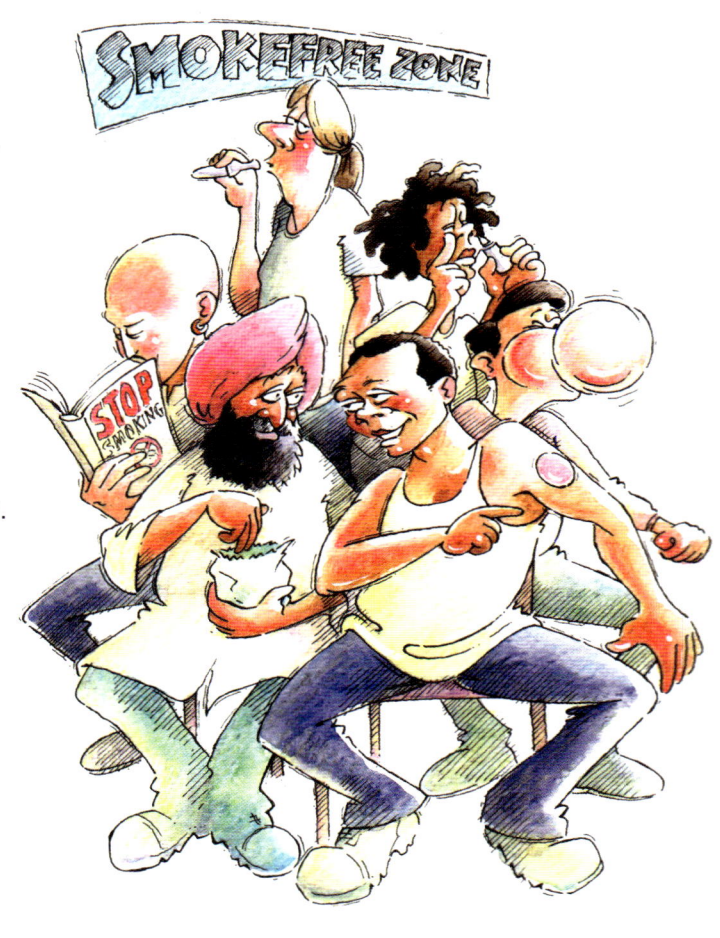

DID YOU KNOW?

- If your lungs were opened up and spread out fully they'd cover an area the size of a tennis court!
- As your heart beats, your blood passes through your lungs and picks up oxygen which it takes to all parts of your body.
- When you exercise your breathing rate goes up because your body needs more oxygen so it can work harder.
- You feel puffed out when your lungs can't supply your body with oxygen quickly enough.
- Regular exercise helps keep your lungs fit and healthy.
- Coughing is a protective reflex – it's the body's effort to get rid of unwanted irritants from the windpipe and the lungs.

- After only 20 minutes of not smoking, your blood pressure and pulse return to normal.
- In just 48 hours, your body is nicotine-free and carbon monoxide (a poison) is cleared from your body.
- And, within 2 to 12 weeks, your blood circulation improves and you'll feel noticeably fitter.
- Best of all, within five years your risk of lung cancer will be much, much lower. And your risk may be halved by the time you reach your tenth year of being tobacco free.

The Choices

Do nothing

Very bad idea.

- Lung cancer was rare until tobacco hit the scene. Some things will not go away in a puff of smoke.
- Lung cancer is the most common type of cancer with over 38,000 new cases in the UK each year. Over one third of all deaths from any cancer are from lung cancer.
- Lung cancer is most common between the ages of 65 and 75 but much younger people will die as well.
- The more cigarettes smoked and the younger the age at which smoking started, the greater the risk.
- Inhalation of tobacco smoke by non-smokers, 'passive smoking', can cause cancer as well.

DIY

What triggers the 'time for a cigarette' habit? Is it:

- When you wake up?
- With the first cup of coffee?
- Talking on the phone?
- Watching TV?
- With an alcoholic drink?
- After a meal?
- While reading?
- When you are stressed?

These are only some examples, and you might have others. Try keeping a diary for a few days to record your smoking patterns. This can help you understand when and why you smoke, and plan what to do instead.

Find an expert

How do I stop? There are a few ways to stop smoking:
- Using effective, free treatments to assist the process.
- Using experienced back-up services and support groups.

Cutting down and cold turkey

The problem with tapering off is that the numbers tend to creep up again, so it is better to stop outright. Make sure you are fully prepared to manage without smoking: many fail because they jump into the task before they are ready. Just quitting with no assistance is hard and is less likely to work in the long term to keep you tobacco free. Consider using other means to help you as well.

Things that can help you

- Prescription and non-prescription aids (see your GP, practice nurse or pharmacist).

Free NHS stop smoking services

You can get a tailored support package (including medications) to help you stop – including one-to-one advice sessions and stop-smoking support groups.

Remember that stopping is better than just thinking about it. People succeed every day – so can you!

Go smoke free

www.nhs.uk/gosmokefree

QUIT PLAN

Whichever you go for, it will be easier with some sort of quit plan.
- Get information. Go online, make a call, visit your surgery or pharmacy. Arm yourself with as much information as possible about the most effective ways available to help you stop and stay stopped.
- Set a day and date to stop. Tell all your friends and relatives, they will support you.
- Like deep sea diving, always take a buddy. Get someone to give up with you. You will reinforce each other's willpower.
- Clear the house and your pockets of any cigarette packets, papers or matches.
- Map out your progress on a chart or calendar.
- Keep the money saved in a separate container.
- Chew on a carrot. It will give you something to do with your mouth and hands.
- Ask your friends not to smoke around you.

NHS Quitline

Tel: 0800 022 4 332
www.nhs.uk/smokefree

NHS Stop Smoking Services

Text GIVE UP, with your post code to 88088 to get localised services

www.givingupsmoking.co.uk

Offers tips, advice and fact sheets to help you quit smoking

www.malehealth.co.uk/smoking

Skin

The Challenge

Show a doctor that thing on your body that's bothering you.

The Reason

There are basically two types of skin cancer.

- Non-melanoma is the most common form of skin cancer. It's commonly found on the forehead, tip of the chin, nose, ears, forearms and hands – basically, all the exposed bits.

- Malignant Melanoma is the more serious form of skin cancer. Although it is much less common, it is on the increase. It often appears as a changing mole or freckle but it can also develop from normal-looking skin.

The Choices

Do nothing

You could also swing a dead cat round your head in a graveyard at midnight.

DIY

Watch out for:
- Size: bigger than the butt end of a pencil (more than 6 mm/quarter inch diameter).
- Colour variety: shades of tan, brown black and sometimes red, blue or white.
- Shape: ragged or scalloped edge and one half unlike the other.

Also watch out for:
- A new growth or sore that does not heal within four weeks.
- A spot or sore that continues to itch, hurt, crust, scab or bleed.
- Constant skin ulcers that are not explained by other causes.

NOT A LOT OF PEOPLE KNOW THIS

- Skin cancer is one of the most common cancers in the UK and not just in women.
- Your lifetime risk as a man of developing skin cancer is one in eight.
- Even cloudy days can deliver 90% of the dangerous UV rays.
- Some football shirts are so thin they let almost all the sunshine through.
- Skin damage remains after your sunburn fades. It builds up under the skin just like rust under bodywork paint and it can come back to haunt you in later years.
- Virtually all the risk comes from overexposure to the sun and sun-beds...

So cover up and close up!

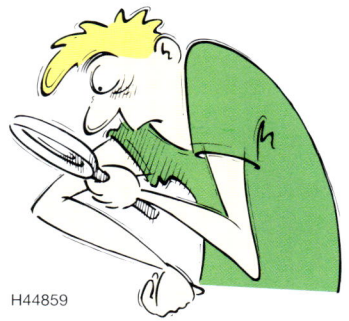

But skin cancer doesn't always have these features. Check your skin regularly and watch out for any changes. Many skin changes are harmless but a quick check with your doctor or pharmacist can save your skin as skin cancer is much easier to treat when it is caught early.

Find an expert

Sunscreens and smokescreens

People get confused over sunscreens and can damage their skin by choosing the wrong sunscreen for them or not using enough. Ask your pharmacist.

Read your sunscreen label and make sure it has both an SPF and a star rating. The SPF or Sun Protection Factor tells you how much protection you are getting from UVB rays.

The star **** rating shows the level of protection against UVA rays. Try to buy a sunscreen that is at least SPF 15+ and has a 4 star rating. Apply it generously half an hour before you go out in the sun and remember to take it with you so you can reapply regularly.

Remember! Wearing sunscreen does not mean that you can stay out in the sun longer. Sunscreen offers some protection, but use it alongside covering up and spending time in the shade to give your skin the protection it needs.

Cancer Research UK
Tel: 020 7242 0200
www.canceresearchuk.org

GET SUN SMART

These five simple steps from Cancer Research UK can help you enjoy the sunshine safely.
- Stay in the shade from 11am to 3pm - summer sun is most dangerous in the middle of the day. Find shade under umbrellas, trees, canopies or indoors.
- Make sure you never burn - sunburn can double your risk of skin cancer.
- Always cover up - sunscreen is not enough. Wear a t-shirt, wide-brimmed hat and wraparound sunglasses (eyes get sun damaged too).
- Remember to take extra care with children - young skin is delicate so keep babies in the shade, especially in the middle of the day.
- Then use sunscreen with a factor of at least 15 - apply it generously 15-30 minutes before you go outside and reapply often

www.malehealth.co.uk/skin

Back

The Challenge

If you've got backache, don't let it become a pain in the arse. Get it sorted.

The Reason

If you've ever suffered from a bad back you'll know just how painful and restrictive it can be – and because other people cannot 'see' the pain you tend to get little sympathy. Bad backs are also one the greatest causes of sickness-related absence from work.

If your job involves lifting heavy objects, sitting at a desk or being immobile for long periods of time, checking your back makes good sense. Chronic back pain can result from bad posture, poor lifting technique or accidental injury.

Being overweight is also a major cause of back problems, not least because it can reduce activity and flexibility, but because it also puts added strain on the muscles, ligaments and bones of the spine. Smoking can also significantly reduce bone strength – which is another good reason for quitting.

Adult bone is constantly being altered and renewed. This needs plenty of calcium. The body can only store this vital mineral in the bone itself, so fresh calcium is needed on a daily basis. The best sources are dairy products such as milk, cheese and yoghurt, but bread is also good, as are fish with edible bones (such as sardines) and green leafy vegetables.

Not only bones can be the cause of back pain. The back is supported by hundreds of different muscles including those that also support the arms, legs and head. All of them can be strained or overworked leaving the spine vulnerable to damage – in fact, most back pain comes from injured muscle or their tendons rather than the spine itself.

The Choices

Do nothing

Your decision, but watch out for straws and camels' backs. You have a staggering 80% chance of developing low back pain at some point in your life. Even stooping to pick up straws may be a problem.

DIY

Most back pain is not due to any serious disease. The acute pain usually improves within days or weeks. Sometimes aches and pains can last for quite a long time. It will settle eventually, but no one can predict exactly when.

- Most people can get back in action

quite quickly, even though they may still have some pain.
- The sooner you get moving and back to normal activities, the sooner you will feel better.
- Rest for more than a day or two can prolong pain and disability.
- How you handle back pain in the early stages is very important to the outcome.
- The longer you remain off work, the less likely you are to return.

When standing for long periods
- Head – keep it up and in line with your spine.
- Shoulders – relax and pull in your shoulder blades.
- Pelvis – keep your hips level while tucking-in your tailbone to line up with your spine.
- Knees – keep slightly bent (not locked).
- Feet – share the weight evenly.

When driving
- Head – use a head restraint at all times.
- Lower back – adjust the seat (or use a small cushion) to give maximum support, and sit well back without slouching.
- Arms – slightly bent.
- Legs – adjust the seat for ease of reaching the pedals (while allowing maximum visibility).
- Take a break – when stopped at the lights, relax by taking your hands off the wheel and bending your legs.

When lifting heavy objects
- Keep your back straight and use your legs to take the strain.
- Know your limits: if it's a two-man job then don't be a one man bad back. It's not always just weight but also the awkward shape or location of a load that can cause problems.
- Make sure you can deal with the shape, clear the area and warn people before you attempt a lift. If the forklifts or trolleys are being used by someone else, wait until they are free – machines are much easier to repair than people.

When using a computer
- VDU – ensure the screen is free from glare and you can clearly see the image (glare can cause headaches).
- Chair – adjust your chair so your eyes are level with the top of the VDU, your forearms are approximately parallel to the desk, and your legs can be moved freely with no pressure from the edge of your seat on the backs of your legs and knees.
- Keyboard – adjust the keyboard so you can rest the hands and wrists in front of the keyboard, and keep your wrists straight while keying (poor wrist posture can also lead to RSI or carpal tunnel syndrome – both extremely painful and debilitating).
- Mouse – again adjust the mouse so it is within easy reach and can be used with the wrist straight while supporting your forearm on the desk.
- Take mini breaks – don't sit in the same position for too long, make

sure you change your posture as often as possible, and take short regular breaks.

Find an expert

If the pain persists or you can't remain in work, you should consult your doctor. He or she will probably advise you to continue with analgesic tablets and keep mobile. You may be advised to have some physiotherapy. Your doctor is unlikely to order further investigations such as x-rays, MRI scans or referral to a specialist unless the pain has persisted for several weeks, is very severe or you have certain signs or symptoms.

Consult your doctor if the following applies to you:

- Unexplained weight loss or fever.
- History of cancer, HIV or long duration use of steroids.
- Difficulty passing or controlling urine.
- Numbness around your back passage or genital area.
- Pain, numbness, pins and needles, or weakness in your leg.
- Unsteadiness on your feet.

X-rays and MRI scans can detect serious back problems, but may be of little use in simple back pain. However, if they don't show anything serious, that's good news. In older people they may show evidence of 'degeneration'. This sounds bad but all it means is normal 'wear and tear'

It is important to stay at work if you can, as this helps you to keep active and recover from the pain. If you do a lot of lifting or have other risk factors in your job, talk to your supervisor or boss and tell them about tasks that you will find difficult to do initially.

A gentle return to full activity is better than weeks of lying in bed with a door under the mattress (in fact, lying flat in a bed for three weeks only makes things worse as it weakens the supporting muscles). Traction (putting huge weights on the legs) belongs in a museum of horrors – it would take a double-decker bus to counter the strength of the back muscles!

Arthritis Care
Tel: 0808 800 4050
www.arthritiscare.org.uk

BackCare
Tel: 0845 130 2704
www.backcare.org.uk

Health and Safety Executive
Tel: 0845 345 0055
www.hse.gov.uk/msd/backpain

National Osteoporosis Society
Tel: 0845 450 0230
www.nos.org.uk

www.malehealth.co.uk/back

BACK TO BASICS; EASING THE PAIN

- Take simple painkillers such as paracetamol or ibuprofen. Always follow the manufacturer's instructions for the correct dose. You should not take ibuprofen if you have a history of stomach ulcer, indigestion, asthma, or kidney disease, or if you are taking warfarin.
- Applying cold to the painful area can numb the pain and limit the effects of any swelling. You can make a cold pack by wrapping ice cubes or a bag of frozen peas in a wet tea towel. Apply the cold pack for no more than 20 minutes at a time. Repeat every 2-3 hours. To avoid burning your skin, make sure you wrap the cold pack in a tea towel before applying it. If you use a packet of frozen peas as an ice pack, you can reuse the same packet several times. However, it's important to remember that you should not eat the contents if they have been defrosted and then refrozen.
- Applying gentle warmth to the painful area can help ease muscle pain. Try a heat pack, hot water bottle or a hot shower. To avoid burning your skin, make sure you don't apply anything too hot and check the skin regularly. You should not apply heat to a new injury – wait at least 48 hours before using heat to ease the pain.
- Bed rest is not helpful for lower back pain – try to continue with your normal activities as far as possible.
- Keep as active as possible and take gentle exercise until the pain eases. Exercises such as walking, swimming and gentle stretching are especially good for back pain and will help to prevent injury in the future.
- Keep a good posture. Try to walk or stand with your head and shoulders slightly back.
- If you are sitting at a desk, make sure that your chair is at the right height for the desk. Your feet should be able to rest flat on the floor, or on a foot rest, with your knees bent at 90 degrees.
- If you are reading, make sure that the book is at eye level so that you do not need to stoop.
- If you are sitting or driving for a long period, make sure you have a seat that supports your back and neck. Take regular breaks to stretch and walk around if possible.
- In bed, use a firm mattress that matches and supports the natural curves of your spine. Lie on your side with your knees bent – avoid lying on your stomach.
- If you are overweight there is extra stress on your back. Losing weight should help reduce your risk of back pain.